Deliciously Low-Carb;

A Culinary Journey

DEBRA TURNEY

Disclaimer

The information provided in this cookbook is for general informational purposes only and is not intended to be a substitute for professional dietary or medical advice. The author and publisher are not responsible for any consequences that may arise from the use of the information contained in this cookbook.

Before making any significant changes to your diet or lifestyle, it is advisable to consult with a qualified healthcare professional or nutritionist. Individual dietary needs vary, and what may be suitable for one person may not be suitable for another.The recipes and meal plans presented in this cookbook are based on the principles of the Low-carb Diet, but it is important to note that individual responses to dietary changes may vary.

7-DAY ATKINS DIET MEAL PLAN

Note: The recipes to the following meals are all included in this book

Day 1

Breakfast: Avocado & Kale Omelet

Lunch: Creamy Pesto Chicken Salad with Greens

Dinner: Horseradish-Crusted Salmon with Crispy Leeks

Day 2

Breakfast: Egg Tartine

Lunch: Barbecue Chicken Kale Wraps

Dinner: Creamy Tomato Salmon

Day 3

Breakfast: Parmesan Cloud Eggs

Lunch: Avocado Ranch Chicken Salad

Dinner: Cheesy Ground Beef & Cauliflower Casserole

Day 4

Breakfast: Tomato-Parmesan Mini Quiches

Lunch: Broiled Cauliflower "Mac" & Cheese

Dinner: Spinach & Artichoke Chicken

Day 5

Breakfast: Banana Pancakes

Lunch: Mozzarella, Basil & Zucchini Frittata

Dinner: Roasted Salmon Caprese

Day 6

Breakfast: Cauliflower Toast

Lunch: Shrimp & Vegetable Soup

Dinner: Shrimp Scampi Zoodles

Day 7

Breakfast: Sausage and Egg Muffin

Lunch: Pickle Sub Sandwiches with Turkey & Cheddar

Dinner: Pork Chops with Balsamic Sweet Onions

<u>About The Author</u>

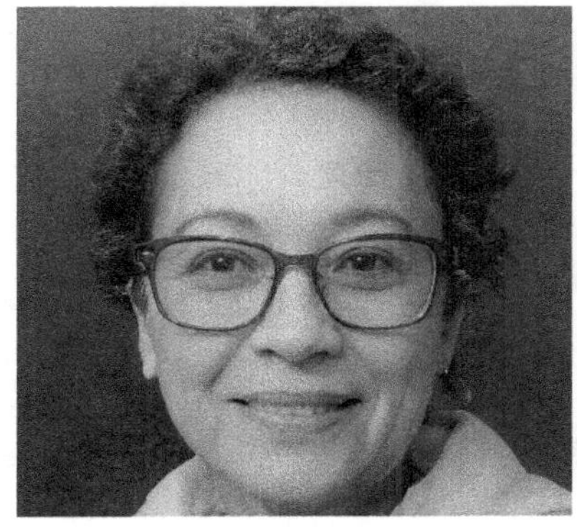

Debra Turney contributes her culinary skills and devotion to this cookbook as a passionate chef who is committed to the practice of mindful living and healthy eating. Debra has dedicated her life to inspiring others to have healthy, balanced lives via her talent for cooking delectable meals that nourish the body and the soul.

Experienced in the culinary arts, Debra's passion for food started in her family's kitchen, where she discovered the healing potential of whole, fresh foods. Her exploration of other cooking methods and cuisines was part of her culinary adventure, but what really won her over was the marriage of nutrition and flavor.

Debra has developed her culinary talents and her awareness of the significant influence that dietary decisions have on one's general well-being as a committed supporter of healthy living. Her dedication to the Low-carb Diet's tenets is a reflection of her faith in the balance that exists between delectable meals and a healthy, active body.

In addition to her passion for cooking, Debra is a loving wife who enjoys treating her family to the benefits of a balanced lifestyle. Here are some thoughtful recipes and tips based on her own experiences developing a fulfilling and well-balanced attitude to food and wellbeing.

Debra Turney extends an invitation to join her on a journey toward a healthier, more energetic version of herself through gastronomy that goes beyond the plate. As you explore the remarkable tastes and nutritional options of the Low-carb Diet, may this cookbook serve as a source of inspiration and delight.

Cheers to enjoying excellent health and the happiness that comes with leading a healthy lifestyle!

<u>Author's note</u>

Welcome to **"Deliciously Low-Carb: A Culinary Journey,"** where flavour meets wellness, and every dish is crafted with your health in mind. In the pages that follow, embark on a culinary adventure that redefines the way we think about low-carb eating.

In a world where dietary choices can often be overwhelming, the low-carb lifestyle stands out as a beacon of balance and vitality. Whether you're a seasoned enthusiast or taking your first steps into the world of reduced carbohydrates, this cookbook is your guide to discovering the joy of nourishing, wholesome meals that are as satisfying as they are nutritious.

The Basics of Low-Carb Eating

We'll start our journey by exploring the fundamentals of low-carb eating, breaking down the misconceptions and providing you with the knowledge to make informed choices. Learn about the benefits of reducing your carbohydrate intake, from improved weight management to enhanced blood sugar control.

A Symphony of Flavors on Every Page

Within these pages, you'll find a collection of meticulously crafted recipes that celebrate the vibrant, diverse world of low-carb cuisine. From hearty breakfasts that kickstart your day to mouthwatering dinners that satisfy your taste buds, each dish is a testament to the richness of flavour achievable within the low-carb spectrum.

More Than a Cookbook, It's a Lifestyle

"Deliciously Low-Carb" is not just a collection of recipes; it's an invitation to embrace a lifestyle that nourishes your body and delights your senses. Through these pages, you'll discover that low-carb eating is not about deprivation; it's about savouring the abundance of fresh, whole foods and enjoying every bite.

So, join me in this culinary adventure, where we celebrate the art of mindful eating and the pleasure of creating meals that contribute to your overall well-being. Let the journey begin—one delicious, low-carb bite at a time.

To your health and happiness,
Debra Turney

TABLE OF CONTENT

INTRODUCTION

A low-carb diet restricts the amount of carbohydrates, or "carbs," which are present in grains, fruit, and starchy vegetables. Diets low in carbohydrates emphasise foods high in fat and protein. There are several kinds or low-carb diets such as; keto ,atkins and paleo

Goal: The main goal of a low-carb diet is to lose weight. Beyond helping you lose weight, several low-carb diets may improve your health by reducing your risk of type 2 diabetes and metabolic syndrome.

Reasons to consider a low-carb diet

Low-carb diet may be your choice if you:
- *Want to reduce weight by restricting some carbohydrates in your diet.*
- *Wish to alter your dietary habits in general.*
- *Savour the kinds and quantities of food that low-carb diets call for.*

Dietary information

A low-carb diet restricts your intake of carbs. The categories of carbs are:
basic
Simple natural sugar such as fructose in fruit and lactose in milk.
Simple refined sugar is one example.
Complex natural foods like beans or entire grains.
Complex Refined foods like white flour.
Grains are a common source of natural carbohydrates.

Complex carbohydrates are generally more slowly absorbed. Additionally, complex carbohydrates affect blood sugar less than refined carbohydrates. They provide fibre as well.
Processed foods frequently contain refined carbohydrates like sugar or white flour. White breads and spaghetti, cookies, cake, candies, and beverages and sodas with added sugar are a few examples of foods high in refined carbohydrates.

Common items in a low-carb diet

A low-carb diet, in general, emphasises meats and some non starchy veggies. Limiting grains, legumes, fruits, breads, sweets, pastas, and starchy vegetables—and occasionally nuts and seeds—is a common practice in low-carb diets.
A low-carb diet typically limits the amount of carbs consumed each day to 0.7 to 2 ounces (20 to 57 grams). These carbs give between 80 and 240 calories. Certain low-carb diets severely restrict carbohydrates in the initial stages of the diet. Over time, those diets permit an increase in carbs.
On the other hand, the Dietary Guidelines for Americans advise that between 45 and 65 percent of your daily calories come from carbohydrates. Thus, carbohydrates would make up between 900 and 1,300 calories per day if you consume 2,000 calories from food or drink.

Benefits

Carbs are the body's primary energy source. Complex carbohydrates are broken down into simple sugars, or glucose, in the process of digestion and then released into the bloodstream. We refer to this as blood glucose.

To enable glucose to enter the body's cells and be used as fuel, insulin is released. Both the muscles and the liver store excess glucose. A portion becomes body fat.

The goal of a low-carb diet is to reduce body weight by encouraging the body to burn fat that has been stored as energy.

Loss of weight

Diets low in carbohydrates, particularly extremely low carb diets, may result in more weight loss in the short term than diets low in fat.

Low-carb diets may cause weight loss for reasons other than just reducing calories and carbohydrates. According to some research, you might lose weight because the additional fat and protein makes you feel fuller for longer. Long-lasting fullness reduces your appetite.

Additional advantages

Low-carb diets that emphasise lean protein, fat, and carb sources may help reduce the risk of heart disease and type 2 diabetes. Actually, practically any diet that aids in weight loss has the potential to lower cholesterol and blood sugar levels.

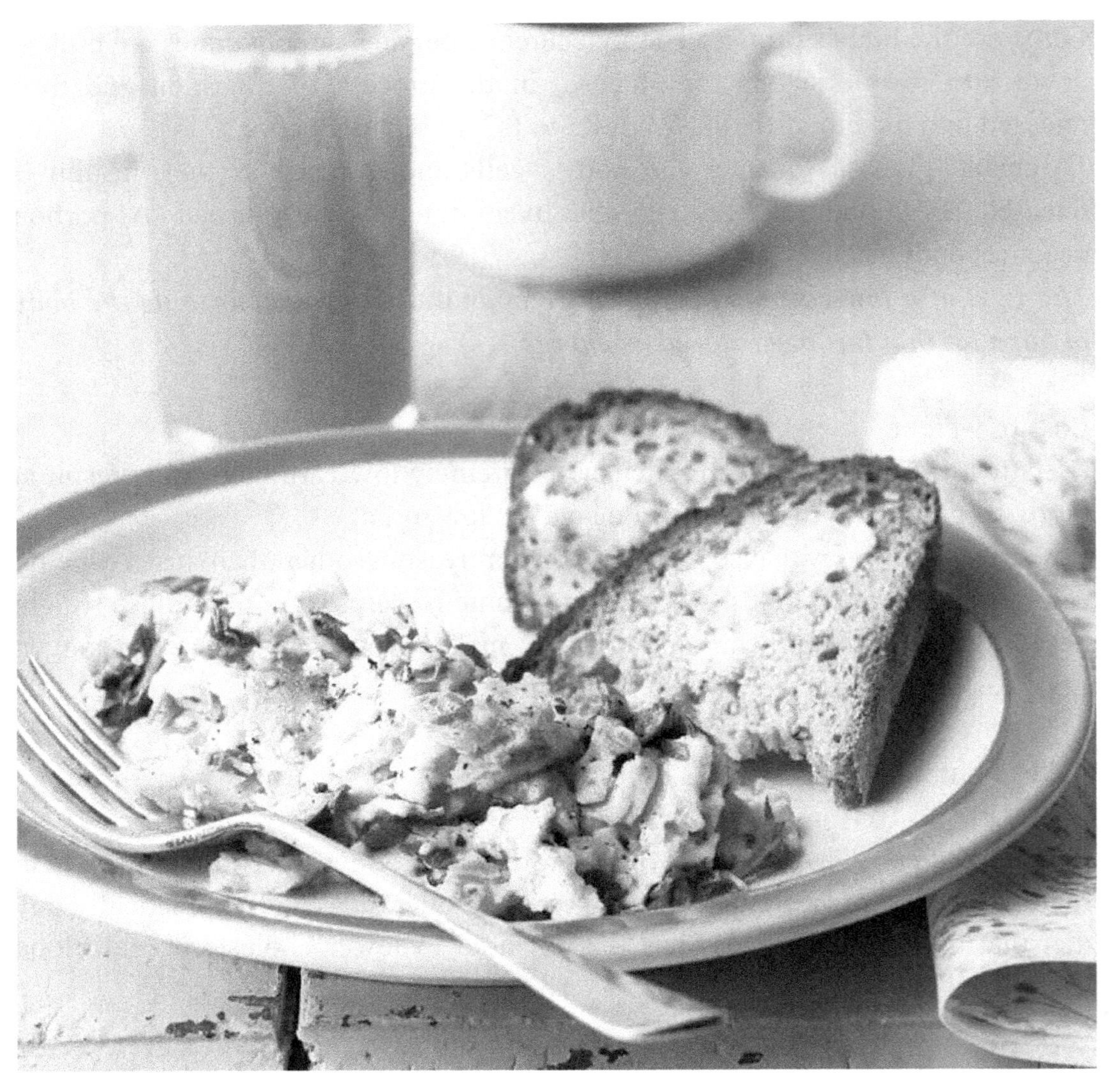

Breakfast

Avocado & Kale Omelet

Prep Time: 10 mins
Cook Time: 10 mins
Servings: 1
Calories: 339

Fat: 28g
Carbs: 9g
Protein: 15g

Ingredients

2 large eggs
1 teaspoon low-fat milk
Pinch of salt
2 teaspoons extra-virgin olive oil, divided
1 cup chopped kale
1 tablespoon lime juice
1 tablespoon chopped fresh cilantro
1 teaspoon unsalted sunflower seeds
Pinch of crushed red pepper
Pinch of salt
¼ avocado, sliced

Directions

1. In a small bowl, beat eggs with milk and salt. In a small nonstick skillet, heat up 1 teaspoon of oil over medium heat. Add the egg mixture and cook for one to two minutes, or until the bottom is set and the middle is still somewhat runny. After flipping the omelette, heat for a further 30 seconds or until it sets. Move to a platter.
2. Combine the kale with crushed red pepper, lime juice, cilantro, sunflower seeds, and the remaining 1 teaspoon oil, along with a small pinch of salt. Arrange the avocado and kale salad on top of the omelette.

Salmon Scrambled Eggs

Prep Time: 10 mins
Cook Time: 10 mins
Servings: 1
Calories: 205

Fat: 13g
Carbs: 2g
Protein :19g

Ingredients

2 large eggs
1 ounce smoked salmon, chopped
2 teaspoons reduced-fat cream cheese
1 scallion, sliced
1 teaspoon capers, rinsed

Directions

1. Lightly beat eggs in a small bowl until mixed. Add capers, cream cheese, scallion, and smoked salmon and stir. Apply cooking spray to a small nonstick skillet and place it over medium heat. Add the egg mixture and simmer for about 3 minutes, stirring frequently, until scrambled

Egg Tartine

Prep Time: 10 mins
Cook Time: 10 mins
Servings: 4
Calories: 184

Fat: 10g
Carbs: 14g
Protein: 10g

Ingredients

1 ½ teaspoons extra-virgin olive oil
4 slices whole-wheat bread, lightly toasted
1 garlic clove, halved
1 medium tomato and/or avocado, sliced
4 large eggs, fried or poached s).

2 tablespoons herbs or microgreens
4 teaspoons capers, rinsed

Directions

1. Apply oil and then garlic to toast. Add the eggs and tomato (or avocado) on top. Add some capers and herbs (or microgreen

Parmesan Cloud Eggs

Prep Time: 25 mins
Cook Time: 25 mins
Servings: 4
Calories: 94

Fat: 6g
Carbs: 1g
Protein: 8g

Ingredients

4 large eggs
Pinch of salt
¼ cup finely grated Parmesan cheese
1 scallion, finely chopped
Ground pepper to taste

Directions

1. Set oven temperature to 450°F. Put parchment paper on the bottom of a large baking sheet. Apply a thin layer of cooking spray.
2. Separate the egg yolks from the whites, setting each yolk aside in a small bowl. In a mixing bowl, use an electric mixer set to high speed to beat all of the egg whites and salt until firm. Using a rubber spatula, gently incorporate Parmesan and scallions into the beaten whites. On the baking sheet that has been preheated, form 4 mounds of the egg-cheese mixture, about 3/4 cup each. Using the back of a spoon, create a well in the centre of each mound.
3. Bake for about 3 minutes, or until the egg whites begin to become a light brown colour. Take out of the oven. Use the spoon to make a new well if the original one has filled in during baking. Carefully place a yolk into every well. Bake for an additional 3 to 5 minutes, or until the yolks are cooked but still runny. Add a little pepper. Serve right away

Tomato-Parmesan Mini Quiches

Prep Time: 25 mins
Cook Time: 25 mins
Servings: 6
Calories: 159

Fat: 8g
Carbs: 5g
Protein: 15g

Ingredients

Nonstick cooking spray
12 4-inch round thin slices lower sodium cooked ham (see Tip)
1 ¼ cups seeded and chopped roma tomatoes
½ cup thinly sliced green onions
1 tablespoon snipped fresh basil or 1 tsp. dried basil, crushed
¼ teaspoon black pepper
⅔ cup finely shredded Parmesan cheese
6 eggs, lightly beaten

Directions

1. Set oven temperature to 350°F. Apply cooking spray to twelve 2 1/2-inch muffin cups.
2. Place ham inside the prepared muffin cups. In each cup, distribute the tomatoes, green onions, basil, and pepper. Add cheese on top. Over the tomato mixture, pour the eggs.
3. Bake for 20 to 25 minutes, or until the tops are puffy and a knife inserted into them comes out clean. Let cool in cups for five minutes. Take out the cups. Garnish with more fresh basil or green onions, if preferred. Serve warm.

Low-Carb Bacon & Broccoli Egg Burrito

Prep Time: 5 mins
Cook Time: 20 mins
Servings: 1
Calories: 259

Fat: 18g
Carbs: 10g
Protein: 15g

Ingredients

1 slice bacon
1 cup chopped broccoli
¼ cup chopped tomato
1 large egg
1 tablespoon reduced-fat milk
1 scallion, sliced
⅛ teaspoon salt
⅛ teaspoon ground pepper
1 teaspoon canola or avocado oil
2 tablespoons shredded sharp Cheddar cheese

Directions

1. In a medium nonstick pan, cook bacon over medium heat for 4 to 6 minutes, rotating once or twice, until crisp. Transfer to a plate lined with paper towels. When the broccoli is tender, add it to the pan and stir-fry it for three minutes. Add the tomato, stir, and then pour into a small bowl.

2. Meanwhile, in another bowl, mix together the egg, milk, scallion, salt, and pepper. After the veggies are done, clean the skillet. Add the oil and turn the heat to medium. Pour in the egg mixture, tilting the pan to cover the bottom. Cook, uncovered, for approximately two minutes, or until the bottom is set. Take a thin, broad silicone spatula and very delicately turn the egg "tortilla." Add the cheese and simmer for a further minute or so, or until it is totally set. Move to a platter. Place the broccoli mixture in the bottom half of the "tortilla" and then cover with the bacon. Form gently into a burrito.

"Egg in a Hole" Peppers with Avocado Salsa

Prep Time: 10 mins
Cook Time: 25 mins
Servings: 4
Calories: 285

Fat: 20g
Carbs: 14g
Protein: 15g

Ingredients

2 bell peppers, any colour
1 avocado, diced
½ cup diced red onion
1 jalapeño pepper, minced
½ cup chopped fresh cilantro, plus more for garnish
2 tomatoes, seeded and diced
Juice of 1 lime
¾ teaspoon salt, divided
2 teaspoons olive oil, divided
8 large eggs
¼ teaspoon ground pepper, divided

Directions

1. Finely chop bell peppers after slicing off their tops and bottoms. Take out and dispose of the membranes and seeds. Cut each pepper into four rings that are 1/2 inch thick.
2. In a medium-sized bowl, mix chopped pepper, avocado, onion, jalapeño, cilantro, tomatoes, lime juice, and 1/2 teaspoon salt.
3. In a big, nonstick pan, heat up one teaspoon of oil over medium heat. Place 4 bell pepper rings on the dish, and then split an egg in the centre of each ring. Add one-eighth teaspoon of salt and pepper for seasoning. Cook for two to three minutes, or until the whites are mostly set but the yolks are still runny. Turn over gently and cook for another minute or two, depending on if you like runny or harder yolks. Repeat with the remaining pepper rings and eggs after transferring to serving dishes.
4. Accompany with the avocado salsa and add more cilantro, if preferred

Cauliflower Toast

Prep Time:10 mins
Cook Time: 35 mins
Servings: 4
Calories: 166

Fat: 11g
Carbs: 8g
Protein: 11g

Ingredients

5 cups cauliflower florets (about 1 pound)
1 cup shredded Cheddar cheese
1 large egg, beaten
¼ teaspoon ground pepper
⅛ teaspoon salt

Directions

1. Preheat the oven to 425 degrees. Using parchment paper, line a single large baking sheet.
2. In a food processor, place the cauliflower. Grate the cheese till it's fine. Move to a bowl that is safe to microwave. Microwave for three minutes on High with a loose cover. Allow to cool a little. After transferring it to a fresh kitchen towel, squeeze off any extra moisture. Go back to the bowl and fully mix in the cheddar, egg, pepper, and salt. Form the cauliflower mixture into eight 3-inch squares on the prepared baking sheet, using approximately 1/4 cup of the mixture for each.
3. Bake for 22 to 25 minutes, or until the toasts are crispy and browned around the edges.

Banana Pancakes

Prep Time: 5 mins
Cook Time: 15 mins
Servings: 2
Calories: 124

Fat: 5g
Carbs: 14g
Protein: 7g

Ingredients

2 large eggs
1 medium banana

Directions

1. Banana and eggs should be blended until smooth.
2. A big nonstick skillet should be lightly oiled and heated over medium heat. Place four heaping tablespoons of batter onto the pan, one for each pancake. Simmer for two to four minutes, or until surface bubbles form and edges seem dry. Take a thin spatula and carefully flip the pancakes over; cook for another one to two minutes, or until the bottoms are golden. After that, move the pancakes to a dish. After using up the leftover batter, give the pan a quick oiling.

Sausage and Egg Muffin

Prep Time: 10 Minutes
Cook Time: 30 Minutes
Servings: 4
Calories: 436.8

Carbs: 2g
Fat: 32.8
Protein: 30.8g

Ingredients

8 ounces Pork Italian Sausage
1/2 pound Ground Turkey
1/2 cup chopped Sweet Red Peppers
8 2/3 large Eggs (Whole)
2/3 tablespoon Parsley (Dried)
1/3 teaspoon Salt
1/4 teaspoon Black Pepper
1/4 teaspoon leaf Dried Thyme Leaves
1/4 teaspoon Paprika
1/8 teaspoon Nutmeg (Ground)
1/8 teaspoon Red or Cayenne Pepper

Directions

1. Turn the oven on to 350°F. Muffin tin with twelve wells: grease it.
2. Sausage and ground turkey should be well combined.
3. Add one egg, diced red bell pepper, parsley, paprika, nutmeg, cayenne, salt, and pepper. Using your hands, combine all the ingredients and mix until well combined.
4. Evenly distribute the sausage mixture (approximately 66 grams per muffin well) across the 12 muffin wells. Making sure there are no holes in the mixture, press the sausage mixture up and slightly over the well rims to form an outer layer.
5. Place one egg into each well and pop them straight into the oven. Bake the eggs for 25 to 30 minutes, or until set. Add cheese and, if preferred, salsa or spicy sauce on top.

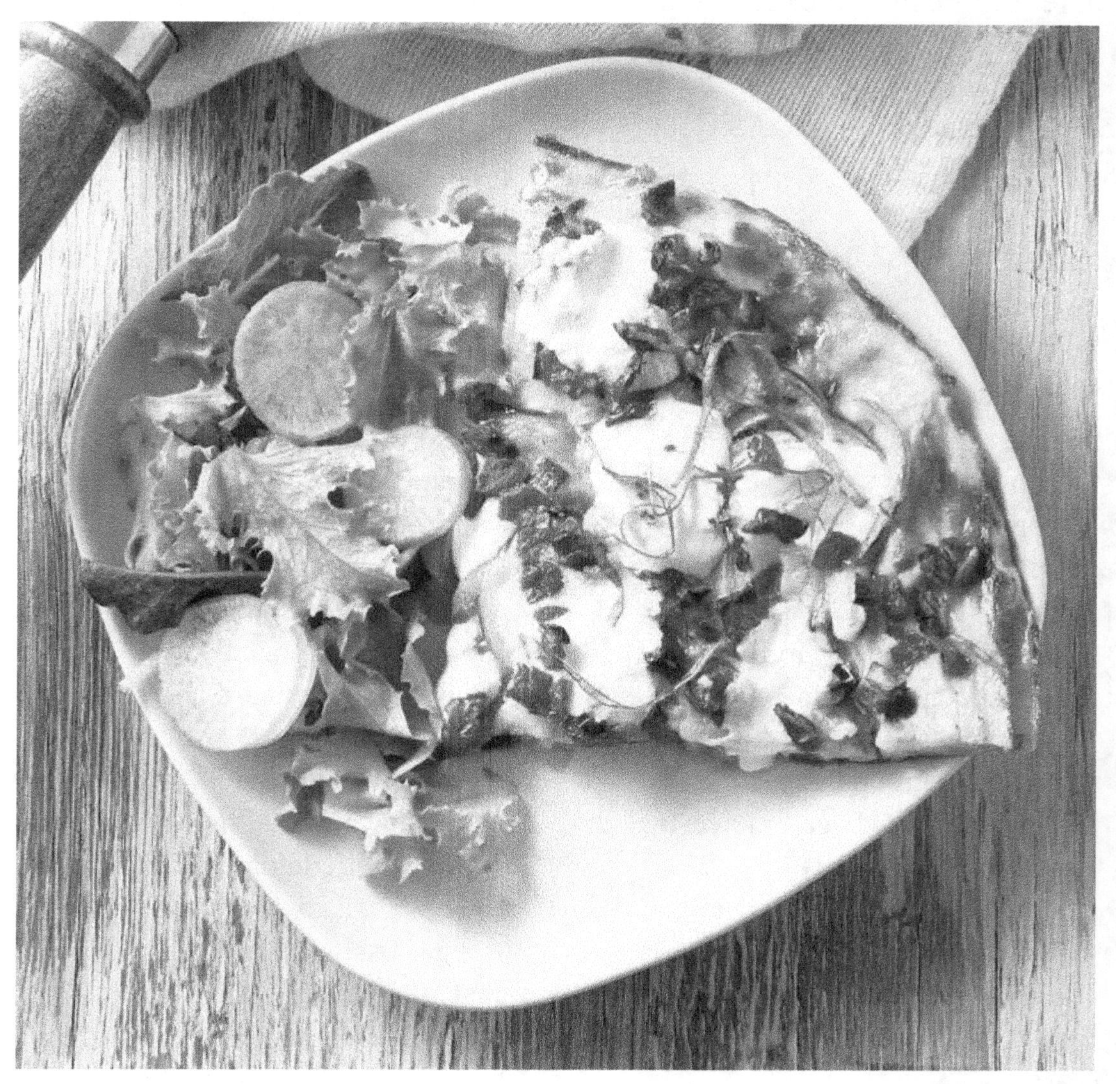

Lunch

Creamy Pesto Chicken Salad with Greens

Prep Time: 30 mins
Cook Time: 30 mins
Servings: 4
Calories: 324

Fat: 20g
Carbs: 9g
Protein: 27g

Ingredients

1 pound boneless, skinless chicken breast, trimmed
¼ cup pesto
¼ cup low-fat mayonnaise
3 tablespoons finely chopped red onion
2 tablespoons extra-virgin olive oil
2 tablespoons red-wine vinegar
¼ teaspoon salt
¼ teaspoon ground pepper
1 5-ounce package mixed salad greens (about 8 cups)
1 pint grape or cherry tomatoes, halved

Directions

1. After putting the chicken in a medium pot, cover it with one inch of water. Heat till boiling. Once the centre is no longer pink, cover, lower the heat to low, and simmer gently for 10 to 15 minutes. When cool enough to handle, transfer to a clean chopping board and shred into bite-sized pieces.
2. In a medium bowl, mix together pesto, mayonnaise, and onion. Toss to coat after adding the chicken. In a large bowl, whisk together oil, vinegar, salt, and pepper. Toss to coat after adding the tomatoes and greens. Arrange the green salad onto four dishes, then place the chicken salad on top.

Barbecue Chicken Kale Wraps

Prep Time: 10 mins
Cook Time: 20 mins
Servings: 4
Calories: 216

Fat: 7g
Carbs: 15g
Protein: 24g

Ingredients

8 small kale leaves or 4 large, cut in half crosswise
1 tablespoon canola oil
1 pound boneless, skinless chicken breast, trimmed and cut into bite-size pieces
¼ teaspoon salt
5 tablespoons prepared barbecue sauce
1 tablespoon rice vinegar
1 ½ teaspoons Cajun seasoning
1 cup thinly sliced red cabbage
1 cup julienned carrots
¼ cup thinly sliced scallion greens

Directions

1. Rinse and pat dry the kale leaves, then trim off any stiff stems or ribs.
2. In a large nonstick skillet, heat the oil over medium-high heat. Add the chicken, season with salt, and heat, tossing often, for 4 to 6 minutes, or until cooked through.
3. In the meantime, combine the vinegar, Cajun spice, and barbecue sauce in a small bowl.
4. After taking the pan off of the burner, pour in the sauce mixture and mix thoroughly. Garnish with scallion greens, cabbage, and carrots and serve within the kale leaves.

Avocado Ranch Chicken Salad

Prep Time: 10 mins
Cook Time: 20 mins
Servings: 6
Calories: 361

Fat: 23g
Carbs: 5g
Protein: 33g

Ingredients

1 ripe avocado, halved and pitted
⅓ cup ranch dressing
2 tablespoons chopped pickled jalapeño
1 tablespoon white-wine vinegar
¼ teaspoon salt
¼ teaspoon ground pepper
3 cups shredded or chopped cooked chicken
¼ cup diced red onion
½ cup diced celery

Directions

1. Put avocado chunks in a food processor. Add vinegar, pickled jalapeño, ranch dressing, salt, and pepper. Process till smooth. To a medium bowl, transfer. Using a rubber spatula, combine the chicken, celery, and red onion. Serve warm or cold

Shrimp & Vegetable Soup

Prep Time: 5 mins
Cook Time: 40 mins
Servings: 6
Calories: 136

Fat: 4g
Carbs: 10g
Protein: 16g

Ingredients

12 ounces fresh or frozen large shrimp, peeled and deveined
4 green onions
2 teaspoons canola oil
2 medium carrots, peeled and thinly sliced
8 ounces fresh shiitake or oyster mushrooms, stemmed and coarsely chopped
1 tablespoon grated fresh ginger or 1 teaspoon ground ginger
2 cloves garlic, minced
2 (14 ounce) cans reduced-sodium chicken broth
2 cups water
1 cup shelled sweet soybeans (edamame)
1 tablespoon reduced-sodium soy sauce
¼ teaspoon crushed red pepper (Optional)
1 cup trimmed sugar snap peas and/or coarsely shredded bok choy
Slivered green onions

Directions

1. If shrimp is frozen, thaw it. After rinsing, blot dry the shrimp with paper towels and leave aside. Slice the entire green onions diagonally into 1-inch-long pieces, being careful to keep the white and green portions apart. Put the green tips aside.
2. Heat the oil in a big, nonstick pot over medium heat. Stir occasionally and simmer for 5 minutes after adding the carrot, mushrooms, and white sections of the green onions. Stir-fry the garlic and ginger for a further minute. To the mushroom combination, add chicken stock, water, soybeans, soy sauce, and crushed red pepper, if preferred. Boil, then turn down the heat. Once the carrot is almost cooked, cover and simmer for about five minutes.
3. Add the bok choy, shrimp, and pea pods to the pot. Reduce heat and bring back to a boil. Cover and simmer for two to three minutes, or until the shrimp turn opaque. Add the tops of the green onions right

before serving. Garnish with slivered green onions, if preferred.

Mozzarella, Basil & Zucchini Frittata

Prep Time:5 mins
Cook Time: 20 mins
Servings: 4
Calories: 292

Fat: 21g
Carbs: 8g
Protein: 18g

Ingredients

2 tablespoons extra-virgin olive oil
1 ½ cups thinly sliced red onion
1 ½ cups chopped zucchini
7 large eggs, beaten
½ teaspoon salt
¼ teaspoon freshly ground pepper
⅔ cup pearl-size or baby fresh mozzarella balls (about 4 ounces)
3 tablespoons chopped soft sun-dried tomatoes
¼ cup thinly sliced fresh basil

Directions

1. Preheat the broiler and place the rack in the upper third of the oven.
2. Apply medium-high heat to a large nonstick or cast-iron pan that is safe for broiling. Stirring constantly, sauté the onion and zucchini for three to five minutes, or until they are tender.
3. In the meantime, beat eggs in a bowl with salt and pepper. Scatter the beaten eggs onto the pan's contents. Cook until almost set, approximately 2 minutes, raising the sides to enable the middle-to-bottom uncooked egg to run below. Put the sun-dried tomatoes and mozzarella on top, then broil the skillet for 1 1/2 to 2 minutes, or until the eggs are just beginning to brown. Allow to stand for a duration of 3 minutes. Sprinkle basil on top.
4. Slide or lift the frittata onto a chopping board or serving dish by

running a spatula around the pan's edge and then beneath. To serve, cut into four pieces.

Cherry Chicken Lettuce Wraps

Prep Time: 10 mins
Cook Time: 20 mins
Servings: 4
Calories: 269

Fat: 12g
Carbs: 11g
Protein: 30g

Ingredients

12 ounces cooked chicken breast, chopped
½ cup sliced celery
¼ cup sliced green onions
¼ cup light mayonnaise
¼ cup plain fat-free Greek yoghourt
2 tablespoons snipped fresh lemon balm or lemon thyme
¼ teaspoon salt
⅛ teaspoon black pepper
8 butterhead lettuce leaves
1 cup quartered fresh dark sweet cherries

¼ cup sliced or slivered almonds, toasted

Directions

1. Mix the cooked chicken breast, green onions, celery, Greek yoghourt, mayonnaise, lemon balm, salt, and pepper in a medium-sized bowl. Place chicken mixture onto leaves of lettuce. Add cherries and almonds on top.

Broiled Cauliflower "Mac" & Cheese

Prep Time: 10 mins
Cook Time: 20 mins
Servings: 8
Calories: 215

Fat: 15g
Carbs: 12g
Protein: 11g

Ingredients

8 cups coarsely chopped cauliflower florets
1 ½ cups reduced-fat milk, divided
2 tablespoons cornstarch
1 teaspoon dry mustard
½ teaspoon ground pepper
¼ teaspoon salt
1 ¾ cups shredded extra-sharp Cheddar cheese
4 ounces cream cheese, cut into 1/2-inch pieces
¼ cup grated Parmesan cheese
Snipped chives for garnish

Directions

1. Arrange the rack in the upper part of the oven. Set the broiler to high temperature.
2. In a big pot, bring the water to a boil. Cook the cauliflower for about five minutes, or until it becomes soft. Drain.
3. Meanwhile, steam 1 1/4 cups of milk in a large broiler-safe skillet over medium heat. In a small bowl, whisk together the cornstarch, dry mustard, and the remaining 1/4 cup milk until smooth. Stir into the heated milk and simmer, whisking continuously, for about two minutes, or until the sauce bubbles and thickens. Take off the heat and whisk in the salt and pepper. Next, whisk in the melted and smooth cream cheese and cheddar. Toss in the cauliflower and stir to coat. Evenly sprinkle the top with Parmesan and broil for three to five minutes, or until browned in spots. Garnish with chives if desired.

Turkey & Cheddar Lettuce Wraps

Prep Time: 5 mins
Cook Time: 15 mins
Servings: 4
Calories: 324

Fat: 22g
Carbs: 3g
Protein: 21g

Ingredients

¼ cup mayonnaise
3 tablespoons chopped dill pickle
2 teaspoons whole-grain mustard
8 large green-leaf lettuce leaves
12 ounces sliced deli turkey
4 ounces sliced deli sharp Cheddar cheese
8 slices tomato

Directions

1. In a small bowl, combine mustard, pickle, and mayonnaise.
2. On a sanitised chopping surface, overlap two lettuce leaves. Dot the lettuce with a liberal 1 tablespoon of the mayonnaise mixture. Add 2 tomato slices, 1 ounce of cheese, and 3 ounces of turkey on top. Roll, then cut in half to form a wrap. Do the same with the remaining ingredients.

Chipotle-Cheddar Broiled Avocado Halves

Prep Time: 10 mins
Cook Time: 20 mins
Servings: 2
Calories: 192

Fat: 17g
Carbs: 9g
Protein: 4g

Ingredients

2 ripe but firm avocados, halved and pitted, skin left on
¼ cup shredded extra-sharp Cheddar cheese
1 small chipotle chile in adobo, minced (about 1 teaspoon), or to taste
1 tablespoon lime juice, plus 4 wedges for serving
Pinch of salt

Directions

1. Turn the broiler on high.
2. Put the halves of avocados on a baking sheet.
3. In a small bowl, thoroughly mix cheese, chipotle, lime juice, and salt. Split the cheese mixture equally between the two avocado halves. For three to five minutes, or until the cheese is bubbling and starting to brown, broil 3 to 4 inches from the heat source. Wait till it's warm, serve with lime wedges.

Pickle Sub Sandwiches with Turkey & Cheddar

Prep Time: 5 mins
Cook Time: 10 mins
Servings: 4
Calories: 186

Fat: 12g
Carbs: 4g
Protein: 12g

Ingredients

8 large kosher dill pickle slices (sandwich stackers)
2 teaspoons mayonnaise
4 ounces deli roast turkey slices
4 (1 ounce) slices Cheddar cheese, halved
8 slices Roma tomato
4 small romaine lettuce leaves

Directions

1. Using paper towels, pat dry the pickle slices. On each of the four pickle slices, spread half a teaspoon of mayonnaise. Add one ounce of turkey, two Cheddar pieces, two tomato slices, and one lettuce leaf on top of each. Add a slice of plain pickles on top.

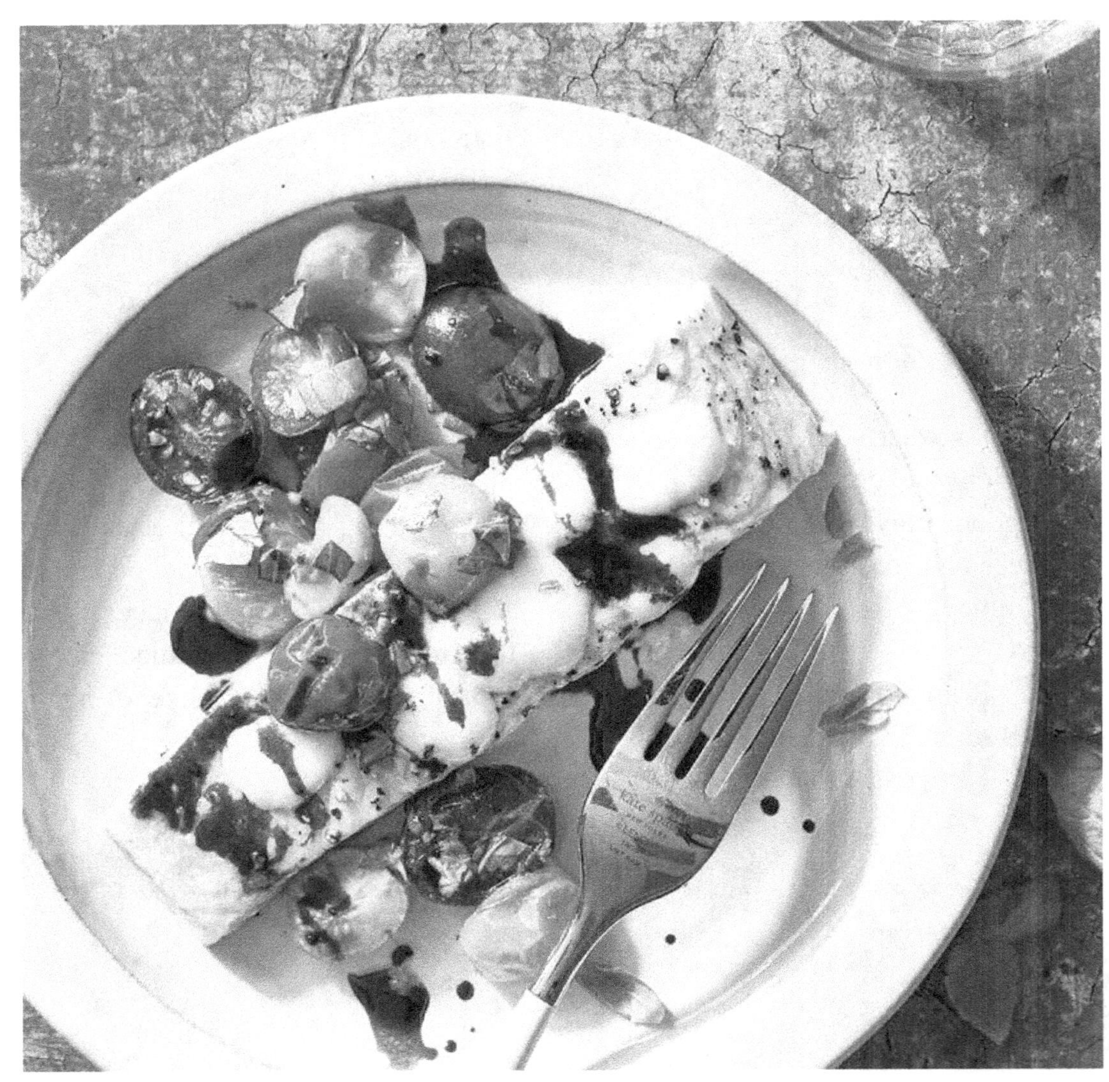

Dinner

Horseradish-Crusted Salmon with Crispy Leeks

Prep Time: 10 mins
Cook Time: 25 mins
Servings: 4
Calories: 326

Fat: 17g
Carbs: 9g
Protein: 29g

Ingredients

1 ¼ pounds salmon fillet, cut into 4 portions
½ teaspoon salt, divided
½ teaspoon ground pepper, divided
2 tablespoons mayonnaise
1 tablespoon prepared horseradish
¼ cup extra-virgin olive oil
1 medium leek, white and pale green parts only, cut into matchsticks
3 tablespoons cornstarch

Directions

1. Turn the oven on to 425°F. Put foil on the rim of a baking sheet.
2. Place the dried salmon on the baking sheet that has been prepared. Add 1/4 teaspoon of pepper and salt to the mixture. In a small bowl, combine the mayonnaise and horseradish, then brush the salmon with it. Roast for 7 to 10 minutes, or until the salmon is opaque throughout.
3. In the meantime, warm up some oil in a big skillet over medium-high heat. Add the leek to the pan after tossing it with cornstarch. Cook for 5 to 8 minutes, stirring occasionally with tongs, or until the leek strands are crispy and golden brown. 4. Transfer to a plate lined with paper towels, then season with the remaining 1/4 tsp. salt and pepper. Top the salmon with the chopped leek and serve.

Creamy Tomato Salmon

Prep Time: 20 mins
CookTime: 20 mins
Servings: 4
Calories: 366

Fat: 21g
Carbs: 10g
Protein: 30g

Ingredients

1 ¼ pounds salmon fillet, skinned and cut into 4 portions
¼ teaspoon salt, divided
¼ teaspoon ground pepper, divided
2 tablespoons olive oil, divided
1 medium zucchini, halved lengthwise and thinly sliced
½ cup chopped onion
⅓ cup dry white wine
1 (15 ounce) can no-salt-added diced tomatoes
2 ounces cream cheese, cut into cubes
1 teaspoon Italian seasoning
½ teaspoon garlic powder
¼ cup chopped fresh basil

Directions

1. Dry off the salmon and then season with 1/8 teaspoon of salt and pepper. In a big skillet, heat up 1 tablespoon of oil over medium-high heat. After adding the salmon, sauté it for 3 to 4 minutes, or until the bottom is browned and it comes out of the pan easily. After flipping, cook the salmon for a further two to three minutes, or until it becomes opaque in the centre. Shift over to a platter.

2. In the meantime, add the onion, zucchini, and remaining 1 tablespoon of oil to the pan. Cook, stirring, for about 3 minutes, or until beginning to soften. Put the heat up to medium-high and pour in the wine. Stir and cook for about 2 minutes, or until the liquid has mostly evaporated. Incorporate the tomatoes, cream cheese, garlic powder, Italian seasoning, and the leftover 1/8 teaspoon of salt and pepper. Bring to a simmer and cook, stirring, for 4 to 5 minutes, or until the cream cheese is melted. Place the salmon back in the pan and turn

it over to coat it in sauce. Garnish
with basil and serve.

Cheesy Ground Beef & Cauliflower Casserole

Prep Time: 10 mins
Cook Time: 30 mins
Servings: 6
Calories: 351

Fat: 23g
Carbs: 11g
Protein: 26g

Ingredients

1 tablespoon extra-virgin olive oil
½ cup chopped onion
1 medium green bell pepper, chopped
1 pound lean ground beef
3 cups bite-size cauliflower florets
3 cloves garlic, minced
2 tablespoons chilli powder
2 teaspoons ground cumin
1 teaspoon dried oregano
1 (15 ounce) can no-salt-added petite-diced tomatoes
2 cups shredded extra-sharp Cheddar cheese
⅓ cup sliced pickled jalapeños
'

Directions

1. Place the rack in the oven's highest third. Turn the broiler on high.
2. In a large broiler-safe skillet, heat the oil over medium heat. Add the onion and bell pepper and simmer, stirring, for about 5 minutes, or until softened. Add the beef and cauliflower, and simmer for 5 to 7 minutes, tossing and breaking up the beef into smaller pieces, until it is no longer pink. Add the chipotle, garlic, chilli powder, cumin, oregano, salt, and chipotle; simmer for one minute or until fragrant. Add the tomatoes with their juices; bring to a simmer and cook, stirring now and again, for another three minutes or more, or until the liquid is reduced and the cauliflower is soft. Take off the heat.
3. After covering the beef mixture with cheese, place sliced jalapeños on top. Broil for 2 to 3 minutes or

the cheese is melted and partially browne

Spinach & Artichoke Chicken

Prep Time: 10 mins
Cook Time: 20 mins
Servings: 4
Calories: 385

Fat: 24g
Carbs: 7g
Protein: 35g

Ingredients

1 (10 ounce) package frozen spinach, thawed
½ cup chopped canned artichoke hearts, rinsed
½ cup shredded Monterey Jack cheese
2 ounces reduced-fat cream cheese, softened
2 tablespoons mayonnaise
1 tablespoon minced shallot
1 large clove garlic, grated
1 pound chicken cutlets
½ teaspoon ground pepper
⅛ teaspoon salt
2 tablespoons extra-virgin olive oil
3 tablespoons grated Parmesan

Directions

1. Turn the broiler on high.
2. Take out as much water as you can from the spinach. Add artichoke hearts, Monterey Jack, cream cheese, mayonnaise, shallot, and garlic to a medium-sized bowl. Mix everything together.
3. After patting the chicken dry, season with salt and pepper. In a sizable cast-iron skillet or other broiler-safe pan, heat the oil over medium-high heat. Cook the chicken in the pan for two to three minutes, or until browned. Cook for a further minute after flipping.
4. Place the spinach mixture over the chicken. Evenly sprinkle on the Parmesan. Put the pan on the broiler and broil for two to three minutes, or until the topping is starting to brown and heated through and an instant-read thermometer placed in

the thickest part of a cutlet reads 165°F

Pork Chops with Balsamic Sweet Onions

Prep Time: 10 mins
Cook Time: 20 mins
Servings: 4
Calories: 246

Fat: 12g
Carbs: 15g
Protein: 20g

Ingredients

4 boneless pork loin chops or cutlets, about 1/2 inch thick, trimmed (1-1 1/4 pounds total)
¾ teaspoon kosher salt
½ teaspoon ground pepper
1 tablespoon extra-virgin olive oil
2 cups thinly sliced sweet onions
1 teaspoon chopped fresh thyme
½ cup unsalted chicken broth
½ cup water
¼ cup golden raisins
3 tablespoons balsamic vinegar
1 tablespoon butter
1 tablespoon chopped flat-leaf parsley

Directions

1. Season pork with sea salt and black pepper. In a big skillet, heat the oil over medium-high heat. Add the pork and heat for about 2 minutes on each side, turning once, until browned. Lower the heat to medium and cook for a further three to five minutes, or until an instant-read thermometer reads 140 degrees Fahrenheit. After moving the pork to a platter, cover it with foil.

2. Add the onions and thyme to the pan and simmer for 1 minute, stirring often. 3. Cook for five minutes while covered, adding water and broth. Uncover and continue cooking, stirring frequently, for approximately 5 minutes, or until the onions are tender and most of the liquid has gone.

4. Scrape up any browned parts as you stir in the vinegar and raisins.

Heat till boiling. Simmer for about 3 minutes, or until thickened. Take off the heat and mix in the butter.

5. Garnish the pork with parsley and serve it with the sauce.

Shrimp Scampi Zoodles

Prep Time: 10 mins
Cook Time: 30 mins
Servings: 4
Calories: 286

Fat: 15g
Carbs: 8g
Protein: 27g

Ingredients

4 to 6 medium zucchini (2 1/4 to 2 1/2 pounds), trimmed
½ teaspoon salt, divided
2 tablespoons butter
2 tablespoons extra-virgin olive oil, divided
1 tablespoon minced garlic
⅓ cup dry white wine
1 pound peeled and deveined raw shrimp (16 to 20 per pound), tails left on, if desired
1 tablespoon lemon juice
¼ cup chopped fresh parsley
¼ teaspoon ground pepper
¼ cup grated Parmesan cheese
Lemon wedges for serving

Directions

1. With a vegetable peeler or spiral slicer, thinly slice the zucchini lengthwise into long, thin strands or strips. Toss the zucchini noodles with 1/4 teaspoon salt after placing them in a sieve. After letting it drain for fifteen to thirty minutes, carefully squeeze off any leftover liquid.
2. In the meantime, place a large skillet over medium-high heat with butter and 1 tbsp oil. Add the garlic and simmer for 30 seconds while stirring. Simmer after adding the wine with caution. Add the shrimp and cook, stirring, for 3 to 4 minutes, or until the shrimp are pink and cooked through. Take off the heat and mix in the remaining 1/4 teaspoon salt, pepper, lemon juice,

and parsley. Move to a sizable bowl and reserve.

3. In the skillet, heat the remaining tablespoon of oil over medium-high heat. Toss gently until the zucchini is heated, about 3 minutes. Over the zucchini, pour the shrimp mixture and toss gently to blend. Serve with a squeeze of lemon and a sprinkling of Parmesan.

Grilled Chicken with Red Pepper-Pecan Romesco Sauce

Prep Time: 10 mins
Cook Time: 30 mins
Servings: 3
Calories: 308

Fat: 20g
Carbs: 8g
Protein: 25g

Ingredients

2 medium red bell peppers
1 medium tomato
1 pound chicken cutlets
¾ teaspoon salt, divided
½ teaspoon ground pepper, divided
½ cup chopped pecans, toasted
1 clove garlic
2 tablespoons extra-virgin olive oil
1 tablespoon red-wine vinegar
¼ teaspoon crushed red pepper
Chopped scallions for garnish

Directions

1. Grill on medium-high heat. For 12 to 15 minutes, grill the tomato and bell peppers, turning them regularly, until they are browned in places and completely blistered. After transferring to a platter, wait five minutes or until the mixture is cool enough to handle.

2. In the meantime, season chicken with 1/4 tsp. salt and pepper. For a total of 6 to 8 minutes, or until an instant-read thermometer placed in the thickest section registers 165 degrees F, grill the chicken, rotating it regularly. Place on a platter, cover with foil, and allow to stand for ten minutes.

3. Take off and dispose of the tomato and peppers' seeds and skins.

To a blender, add the peppers, tomato, pecans, garlic, oil, vinegar, crushed red pepper, and the remaining 1/4 teaspoon of pepper and 1/2 teaspoon of salt. On high, puree for one minute, or until well blended. If preferred, garnish the chicken with scallions and serve it with the sauce.

Broiled Cod with Tomatoes & Herbed Mayonnaise

Prep Time: 5 mins
Cook Time: 15 mins
Servings: 4
Calories: 226

Fat: 11g
Carbs: 4g
Protein: 26g

Ingredients

¼ cup mayonnaise
3 tablespoons chopped herbs such as basil, tarragon or cilantro
1 teaspoon garlic powder
½ teaspoon onion powder
½ teaspoon salt, divided
½ teaspoon ground pepper, divided
1 ¼ pounds cod, cut into 4 portions
2 medium tomatoes, sliced

Directions

1. Set the rack four inches away from the heat source and turn the broiler on high. Put foil on a baking sheet.
2. In a small bowl, stir together mayonnaise, herbs, garlic powder, onion powder, ¼ teaspoon salt, and ¼ teaspoon pepper. Remaining ¼ teaspoons of salt and pepper should be applied on both sides of the cod. Arrange the fish on the baking sheet that has been prepared, then coat each piece with the mayonnaise mixture. Add slices of tomato on top. Broil for 8 minutes.

Tarragon Scallops on Asparagus Spears

Prep Time: 5 mins
Cook Time: 25 mins
Servings: 4
Calories: 253

Fat: 12g
Carbs: 14g
Protein: 27g

Ingredients

1 ¼ pounds fresh or frozen sea scallops
1 cup water
1 pound asparagus spears, trimmed
2 medium lemons
½ teaspoon ground pepper
¼ teaspoon salt
1 tablespoon extra virgin olive oil
3 tablespoons vegetable oil spread
1 tablespoon chopped fresh tarragon or 1 teaspoon dried tarragon

Directions

1. If scallops are frozen, thaw and set aside. In a large nonstick skillet over medium-high heat, bring the water to a boil. Add the asparagus, return to a boil, lower the heat, cover, and simmer for 3 to 5 minutes, or until the asparagus is crisp-tender. Thoroughly drain, transfer to a serving dish, and gently cover to maintain warmth.
2. Segment one of the lemons. Shred 1 teaspoon of the leftover lemon peel finely. Extract two teaspoons of lemon juice.
3. Dry the scallops using paper towels. Season scallops with salt and pepper.
4. Dry-wipe the skillet. Oil should be heated to a medium temperature. In two batches, sauté the scallops for 3 minutes, then flip them over and cook for an additional 2 minutes, or until they are golden brown and slightly opaque in the centre. On top of the asparagus, arrange the cooked scallops.
5. To the skillet, add the vegetable oil spread, tarragon, lemon peel, and

1 tablespoon of lemon juice. Simmer for one minute to slightly thicken. If preferred, add the remaining lemon juice. Pour over the scallops. Accompany with wedges of lemon.

Roasted Salmon Caprese

Prep Time: 10 mins
Cook Time: 30 mins
Servings: 4
Calories: 291

Fat: 18g
Carbs: 5g
Protein: 26g

Ingredients

1 ½ teaspoons extra-virgin olive oil
1 clove garlic, grated
½ teaspoon salt, divided
½ teaspoon ground pepper, divided
2 cups quartered cherry tomatoes
1 pound salmon fillet, skin removed, cut into 4 pieces
1 ounce pearl mozzarella balls, halved
¼ cup thinly sliced basil

Directions

1. Set oven temperature to 425°F. Apply cooking spray to a large baking sheet with a rim.
2. In a small bowl, stir together oil, garlic, and 1/4 teaspoon each of salt and pepper. Toss in tomatoes to coat.
3. Place the fish on half of the baking sheet that has been prepped. Add the final 1/4 teaspoon of each seasoning to the mixture. Place chunks of mozzarella over the tops of the fillets. Transfer the tomato mixture to the opposite side of the pan. Bake for 8 to 10 minutes, or until the tomatoes are soft and the salmon is just cooked through. After adding basil to the tomato sauce, serve it with the salmon.

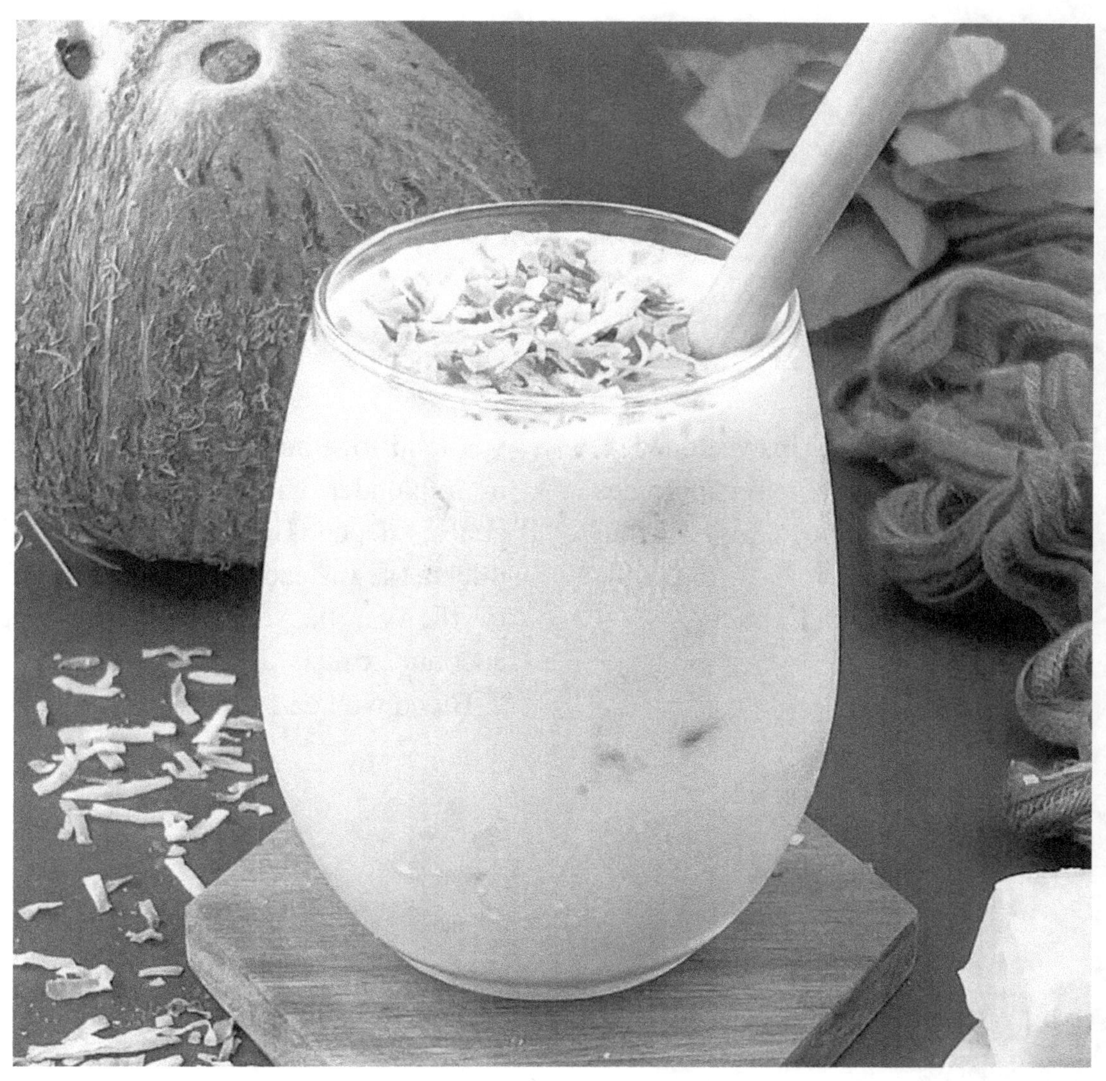

Smoothie

Coconut Protein Shake

Prep Time: 5 Minutes
Cook Time: 0 Minutes
Servings: 1
Calories: 158.7

Fat: 5.6g
Carbs: 1.3g
Protein: 24.4g

Ingredients

1 cup Coconut Milk Unsweetened
1 ounce Protein Technologies International ProPlus Soy Protein Isolate
1/2 teaspoon Vanilla Extract

Directions

1. Blend together all the ingredients in a blender with one to four ice cubes, depending on the desired thickness. Instead of or in addition to the vanilla, think about using coconut extract.
2. Blend well and serve.

Coconut-Vanilla Shake

Prep Time: 5 Minutes
Cook Time: 0 Minutes
Servings: 4
Calories: 73.4

Fat 1.7g
Carbs: 0.9g
Protein: 12.9g

Ingredients

1 1/2 cups Coconut Milk Beverage, plain, unsweetened
2 scoops Vanilla Whey Protein
1/2 teaspoon Vanilla Extract

1. Blend 2 cups of ice cubes, protein powder, coconut milk, and vanilla in a blender until smooth and creamy. Add 1/4 tsp of coconut extract if you'd like more taste. Without adding any more NC, MCT oil gives this smoothie an extra creamy texture. Try adding one tablespoon before blending.

Directions

Chocolate Hazelnut Smoothie

Prep Time: 3 Minutes
Cook Time: 0 Minutes
Servings: 2
Calories: 315.3

Fat: 22g
Carbs: 2.7g
Protein: 26.2g

Ingredients

2 scoops Chocolate Whey Protein
1/2 cup Heavy Cream
1/4 cup tap water
2 tablespoons hazelnut syrup, sugar free
1 cup municipal tap ice cubes

Directions

Note on ingredients: I recommend using a chocolate whey protein powder with 1 net carb and 25 g protein per scoop for this recipe.

1. In a blender with about a cup of ice, combine the protein powder, cream, water, and syrup; process until smooth.
Transfer to two glasses. If desired, top with a cinnamon sprinkle.

Snickerdoodle Smoothie

Prep Time: 5 Minutes
Cook Time: 0 Minutes
Servings: 2
Calories: 161.4

Fat: 5g
Carbs: 3.7g
Protein: 25.1g

Ingredients

1 cup Coconut Milk Beverage, plain, unsweetened
1 scoop (1 scoop= 31 g) Quest Vanilla Milkshake Protein Powder
1 teaspoon Cinnamon, ground

Directions

1. Mix all ingredients until extremely smooth, excluding ice. Enjoy after blending or pouring over 1/2 cup of ice.

Keep in mind that you may use any sugar-free milk—like almond, soy, or cashew in place of the coconut.

Vanilla-Spinach Shake

Prep Time: 5 Minutes
Cook Time: 0 Minutes
Servings: 1
Calories: 174

Fat: 3.9g
Carbs: 2g
Protein: 27.4g

Ingredients

1 1/2 cups Almond Breeze Unsweetened Vanilla Milk
1 cup Spinach
1 teaspoon Vanilla Extract
1 ounce or scoop Vanilla Whey Protein

Directions

1. After adding two glasses of ice to a blender, add all the ingredients and process until smooth. You can adjust the sweetness by using small amounts of powdered stevia or drops of stevia, depending on your own choice.

Dear Valued Reader,

I hope you've enjoyed exploring the culinary delights within the pages of **"Deliciously Low-Carb: A Culinary Journey,"** Your satisfaction is of utmost importance to me, and we would greatly appreciate your feedback to help us continue improving and providing valuable content.

If you've found inspiration in the delectable recipes, insightful meal plans, and practical tips shared in this cookbook, I'd like to invite you to share your thoughts by leaving a review. Your honest opinions can assist other readers in making informed decisions and contribute to the ongoing success of our community.

Here are a few questions to guide your review:

1. What recipes did you find most enjoyable or helpful?
2. How has the cookbook influenced your approach to the Low-carb Diet or healthy living?
3. Were the meal plans and tips practical and easy to implement into your routine?
4. Do you have any favourite features or aspects of the cookbook that stood out to you?

Your feedback is invaluable to me, and I appreciate you taking the time to share your thoughts. Thank you for being a part of our journey toward healthier and more delicious living.

Thank you for your support!

Warm regards,

DEBRA TURNEY

I'm sure you don't intend to stop your cooking journey here, why don't you hop on a ride with me and unlock the secrets to healthy living while perfecting your craft in the kitchen. **INTRIGUED?**

SCAN the QR code below to check out other books by me !